SUCCESSFUL AGING

BLUEPRINT

A STEP-BY-STEP GUIDE
TO RECLAIMING
YOUR HEALTH
AND DEVELOPING
A RESILIENT MINDSET
AFTER AGE 45

ART MCDERMOTT, CSCS CISSN

FROM THE *SUCCESSFUL AGING ACADEMY*

TABLE OF CONTENTS

ABOUT THE AUTHOR

Art McDermott CSCS CISSN

Founder and Chief Motivational Officer at the Successful Aging Academy

Speaker | Author | Over 45 Advocate | Successful Aging Rebel

Art McDermott is a Certified Nutritionist, and has been a Certified Strength and Conditioning Specialist for 30 years.

He has spent years in the private and corporate wellness arenas; teaching, public speaking, implementing corporate fitness programs, consulting and overseeing curriculum development.

Art's mission to the help individuals ages 45 and older to take charge of their coming decades mentally and physically, using a straightforward sequential approach.

Art has owned several training facilities specializing in personal training, nutrition, fitness/physique transformations, 'over 45' and senior training, as well as sports preparation.

Career highlights:

- Adjunct Professor – University of Massachusetts, Lowell. College of Health Sciences.
- Serial Entrepreneur & Lifetime Learner
- 6 Time NCAA All-American in Track & Field, and a member of multiple US National and International Teams
- Proud Dad

Current Published Books:

- *"Move More, Save More – Guidelines for Boosting Profits, Morale and Retention with Corporate Wellness"*
- *"Boomer Blueprint – A Step-by-Step Guide to Longevity, Anti-Aging and Fitness for Baby Boomers"*
- *"The Red Wine Diet – Enjoy Life. Lose Fat."*

ACKNOWLEDGEMENTS

Trying to thank all those who have influenced and motivated me along my path would be difficult, to say the least.

However, in the many times when I doubted myself, facing challenges both physical and situational, there was one who never wavered in her support of my efforts.

My mother also just so happens to be a model for how to stay strong, stay focused, endure, stay sharp and generally age beautifully and successfully.

Thank you Pat Gill.

PROLOGUE

It's time to start thinking about our health and mindset in a completely new way.

The vast majority of people we know do not sit around and ponder what they might be able to do today to improve their health.

But I believe it's about time we do exactly that.

What if we gave our mental and physical health the same focus and attention as we did our income?

What if we viewed getting and staying healthy as an immutable obligation, on par with paying the mortgage or protecting our children?

My question is: Why wouldn't we?

The minute we decide to ignore our health (both mental and physical) we have made a conscious decision to put that burden upon someone else – usually other members of our own family, or even society as a whole.

Maybe not right away, but eventually.

The medications, the surgery, the loss of independence, the simple inability to fulfill daily obligations like transportation, social interactions...mental calculations and more.

Imagine no longer being able to help with family advice and decisions. Instead, the conversation turns to "well, mom is certainly not getting around like she used to" or "There's no way dad is going to be able to handle that (any physical household task) anymore."

Think this can't happen? Think this is too farfetched?

Think again.

We are all making decisions TODAY that will determine the quality of life we will have in 10, 20 or 30 years from now.

So, how much thought are you putting into those decisions?

There are lots reasons and excuses we put forward for avoiding the work required to make a positive change. (And we will destroy every one of these reasons in this book!)

Yet, every day we see examples of people who have successfully made massive lifestyle changes.

So, this begs the question...

What is the difference between the individual who steps up and makes a radical lifestyle change, and the one who never gets moving in the right direction?

This could apply to quitting cigarettes, losing weight, breaking a destructive habit, quitting drinking, removing sugar from the diet, etc.

Do the people who do this successfully have some secret storage of super will power? Absolutely not. (In fact, we'll look at the fallacy of relying on 'will power' to evoke change later on.)

Contrary to what you might believe, these people did NOT wake up one day out of the blue and "change".

The seeds of change had been festering for a long time prior; perhaps for years and years.

A buildup was occurring.

They thought everything through, either on a conscious or unconscious level, until they were ready.

Without even knowing it, their success stories had a system in place.

Their hurdles and obstacles had been mentally addressed *PRIOR* to any true change being made.

And you can do the same. No matter what your goal is!

The fact is most people simply need their own personal system for addressing these hurdles and obstacles.

Things like: a support system, replacement behaviors, a pattern of interruption or disruption, positive reinforcement, and more.

This is EXACTLY what we will be spelling out for you here.

Imagine having the confidence to face any bad habit, any personal, mental, or physical goal and know *BEFOREHAND* that you can succeed.

What could stop you?

Nothing.

The reason most people fail when it comes to things like breaking a bad habit, losing weight, going to the gym, etc. is the complete lack of a habit change system to rely on.

Their plan becomes wishful thinking...nothing more.

By the end of this book...and as part of the Successful Aging Academy (SAA) program, you will have a repeatable, reliable system you can turn to when faced with any personal change you need to make.

Before we begin, however, it's necessary to expose the true enemies of this entire process.

Let's do it!

CHAPTER 1

IDENTIFYING THE TRUE ENEMIES AND DEFINING CORE CONCEPTS

There are some consistent themes you should notice throughout this book. They are, in no particular order; inertia, disruption, expectations, acceptance vs obligation, accountability, planning, and readiness.

These may seem like odd topics for what is essentially a life coaching/wellness/fitness book.

But based on my experience helping thousands of clients, these powerful concepts make the difference between someone taking control of their health...or becoming an unhealthy statistic.

Let's define them.

Inertia refers to what happens when life gets in the way of our health. We get busy. We have a steady flow of obligations and an ever-increasing demand upon our time and energy.

Our health slowly gets pushed to life's back burner.

That's when inertia sets in.

Changing our lives to incorporate exercise, fixing our nutrition and improving our mental approach to aging becomes a huge challenge.

In many cases, it takes a specific event to alter this course of action – or lack of action. Such an event might be a medical scare or even the unexpected death of someone in our own age group; otherwise known as the "wake-up call".

The motive for change can also be less traumatic, but just as effective.

Motivation can occur simply from catching your reflection in the mirror on just the right day and in just the right light, revealing someone unrecognizable. Perhaps you wake up one day as a peri-menopausal female who is "suddenly" twenty, thirty, or more pounds overweight.

Perhaps, as a male, you see someone in the mirror bearing no resemblance to the image you have in your mind as to how you *thought* you looked.

That one reflection starts the wheels in motion, because you realize the alternative is unacceptable for you.

If only you had a system…

Then comes our **Expectations**. In my experience, most individuals past age 50 set their goals far too low by embracing thoughts such as 'act your age', 'slow down and take it easy', and 'I'm too old to (fill in any challenging activity or change).'

Many of us don't *expect* to be strong and lean ever again!

This is just plain wrong.

I believe it is possible to set your expectations higher, and demand just a bit more from yourself than you thought you could.

It simply requires a step-by-step process.

Once your mind creates the vision of who you want to be, together we will find your unique path to make it happen.

Acceptance is the enemy!

Once you have accepted yourself as you are, with little plan for change…you will get just that. "I'm fifty-five. I can't do that stuff anymore."

This is a load of garbage.

Resources like the Successful Aging Academy©
are designed to alter these limiting expectations, destroy
acceptance of an inevitable downward spiral, and provide
the plan to get to where you really want to be.

Using an example from earlier; if you have ever had
a mortgage, you fully understand the obligation that it
entails. You *MUST* pay that mortgage each and every
month. Without fail.

If you don't, there are serious consequences. You could
very likely lose your home. At best, your credit will be
destroyed.

We need to view the preservation of our mental and
physical capabilities in the exact same way!

This is an irrefutable, uncompromising obligation.

If you neglect your brain health, allow a mental issue
to fester or, more commonly, allow your physical health to
deteriorate, there will be consequences.

Therefore, we have an **obligation** to ourselves and those
around us to fulfill these needs with the same urgency as we
address our finances.

The SAA factors in this obligation are in the form of
accountability. You will oversee the construction of your
own personal support and accountability coaching program.

You are the general contractor on the "Ideal You Project"!

Accountability = Obligation = Success.

With this type of structure in place, your odds of success – no matter what your goal is – increases 10 fold.

It's been said that many people don't think much about their health until they lose it. Sadly, this is all too true.

Your doctor announces to you that your fasting glucose test shows you to be pre-diabetic.

How do you react? With panic or a shrug?

You can just take a pill, and your blood sugar will go back to normal. Right?

WRONG!

It cannot become the 'new normal' in your life to let filling a prescription take the place of ACTIVE control of your health.

Pre-diabetes is 100% reversible. 100%! Don't let the ads on TV convince you otherwise. They will try to convince you that this is some 'condition' that just happens to strike you. Purely random right?

Wrong.

This condition is 100% under our control.

Now, prediabetes may not be your hurdle. It could be any number of things that we will work on together to pinpoint. And now is as good a time as any to say that the Successful Aging Academy does not refer to these various hurdles as "hurdles" at all.

Let's face it. They are rocks. Big Rocks.

Your Big Rock is that thing…that one thing in your life that, if you were to overcome it, would change everything. You would become unstoppable.

Together we'll define your Big Rock(s). Then we'll create a plan to reduce each Big Rock to dust…and watch it blow away, leaving behind nothing but an ideal version of you.

Planning

If you have no plan, you have nothing.

I have worked with many people who were – by financial standards – quite successful. Yet, they found it virtually impossible to create a plan to live long enough to enjoy their own financial success.

This defies logic.

Without health, everything else is secondary. If you fail to take care of your health, your ability to enjoy the life you have built, and to help those around you, is seriously compromised.

While conducting research for this book, I examined several of the more popular home-based fitness DVD products currently on the market and saw one recurring – and serious- flaw.

While these products may be wonderful for a youthful population, folks over fifty are very likely to become injured attempting the same training.

This fact is another driving force behind the Successful Aging Academy©. Executing the right movements, in the right amount, with the proper frequency is very important.

This is also known as having a plan.

Everyone needs a plan; one that is tailored to them and to their individual needs.

Understanding standards or 'norms' for your age group, and understanding the little things you can and should be addressing, allows you to determine the *right* program for you. A generic program, usually tailored to that younger audience, will NOT help you, and can actually cause you severe injury.

The other part of planning that is largely ignored involves nutrition.

Without some planning, you will end up making terrible dietary decisions. It's unavoidable.

Poor meal planning – such as going for too long between meals so your blood sugar falls to very low levels – results in an almost overwhelming desire to eat just about anything readily available.

Anything.

This is a very simple example, and one easily rectified with some basic planning.

In fact, I will go so far as to say that **a lack of planning is the #1 reason many people fail with their nutritional approach**.

Now, my favorite theme…and likely the most powerful for you to recognize.

Disruption.

Much like Uber has completely disrupted the ride hailing world, disrupting our own patterns of behavior and beliefs can be life-altering…in a great way.

This is the crux of what we will now discuss.

When done properly, one's disrupting habits and patterns that have been engrained for years, can suddenly disappear.

These are likely the patterns that are literally killing us.

So I ask that you be open to the possibility of throwing out the window at least one or two of your existing daily or weekly patterns, and replacing them with new patterns; patterns that will positively impact your quality of life, as well as its length.

We will show you exactly how to do this.

Once we become aware of these themes in our lives, new behaviors will emerge, new beliefs take the place of old ones, and prior low expectations no longer interest us.

Successful aging begins.

As a member of the Successful Aging Academy you will be asked to pinpoint your "disruption"; the behavior you deliberately chose to execute which will completely upend a negative pattern that is destroying your mental or physical health.

You may know what your disruption is right now. Maybe it popped into your head with no prompting. If not, no worries. We will work together to pin down this behavior.

You may not think of yourself as a disrupter…but you will.

Because, without disruption you are left with a cycle of 'sameness', that may eventually kill you, or at least shorten your life. With it, you will become a powerful voice arguing against 'normal' aging.

This is the rebel refusing to go along quietly.

The primary tool of this disruption can be found in the core system behind the Successful Aging Academy…the HC45 Program. This stand for: Habit Changes for those over 45.

This science based system will allow you to take on any bad habit, any destructive tendency, and break it down into its smaller components, and then crush it.

The power of this change agent type of system cannot be understated.

Most people truly want to change…if they only knew how. They have never had the power of ANY system behind them before. Never mind something created SOLELY to pinpoint and destroy the habits conspiring to ruin their lives and crush their quality of life.

The next key theme is one of **Readiness.**

One of the core mantra of SAA is one simple question:

Are you ready?

I am not trying to sound negative here, but if you are over age 45, it is likely you have faced some sort of "challenge" or serious life crisis.

...a new job

...an unexpected move

...a health scare

...the loss of someone close to you

You get the idea.

The point is, when these events occur, are you ready to deal with them?

Do you have the mental, physical or spiritual reserves to take them in stride?

A simple example...

If you were suddenly faced with a significant surgery... would you be ready... at all levels?

This actually happened to me. I will share that story with you in a later chapter.

Unexpected. Sudden. Life-changing.

You have no choice but to deal with it. And how well you handle any challenge depends upon whether or not you were READY!

Finally, I hope you realize as you go through this book, that you *CAN* do this.

You CAN make the personal change you desire to, no matter how many times you may or may not have failed in the past.

It is not your will power or self-discipline that is at fault here. You have simply been using the wrong system...or not using a system at all.

Minor alterations to your "system" can change everything!

All of the above information actually represents the very foundation of the Successful Aging Academy©.

Let's be clear on what we are talking about.

The SAA 'curriculum' is built around you and your re-creation. The result is called the "Ideal YOU Project".

Think of it as your final exam.

Every step defined. Every trouble spot erased.

You should know that these core concepts are discussed in more detail through the podcasts, blogs and programs found within the academy.

www.successfulaging.academy

We want your new "mantra" to go like this:

I am mobile and strong.

I am resilient.

I embrace action.

I dictate my own future.

I disrupt the status quo.

I am a successful aging rebel.

I am ready

CHAPTER 2

THE PURPOSE BEHIND THIS BOOK

In short, the primary purpose of writing this book is to provide a starting point for people just like you, who realize they have to do *something*.

What about the formation of the Successful Aging Academy?

Call this bold, but we are on a mission to influence every individual between ages 45 through 65 who has let any aspect of their health suffer. We want to create an entire generation of successful aging rebels!

This means mentally, physically, socially and spiritually.

You want to make a change, but maybe have either tried and failed in the past, made specific plans, but never followed through or simply have come to the inevitable conclusion that your status quo may very well be shortening your life.

Many people I work with say, "And now what? What's my first step?"

As with any topic or situation, if there is simply too much information available, people become overwhelmed and end up taking no action at all.

Any salesman will tell you that if you give a consumer too many choices, they become incapable of making a clear decision and generally walk away. It is easy for all of us to become overwhelmed with the amount of data and new information coming out virtually every day, telling us what's good for us and what's bad for us.

Few areas of study have more misinformation than the areas of health, wellness, and nutrition.

As a fitness professional, I find this extremely frustrating.

I often have people coming to me saying "Yes, but I read this, and I also read just the opposite. I'm not sure what to do." One week something can be good for you, and the next study comes out saying it's bad.

So what do people do?

They don't do anything.

Information overload or 'paralysis by analysis' can halt you in your tracks before you even start. I've done my best to cut through all that for you. I want to provide a simple step-by-step process that allows you to take control of your health and your life – the way you were meant to.

Many of the recommendations and much of the information contained in this book are based on a few simple premises.

You are physically and mentally capable of significantly more than you believe you are.

Our bodies and minds are remarkably strong and resilient.

Therefore, our purpose is to put this mindset to use, and seize a chance to retain or regain our definition of success in any number of categories.

Take the simple category of physical fitness.

Physical activity is what we were designed to do.

So…with this in mind, let's put to rest the "I'm too old" excuse right off the bat.

As soon as you buy into the "I'm too old" thing, the mental side of the battle is compromised.

DON'T let that happen.

With the increase in our life spans that we've seen over the last century, also comes an increase in the number of our active years.

This just makes sense.

So now we can see that we have a physiological obligation to remain vital and active for a longer period of time.

Heck, studies show we can gain significant strength levels well into our 90's.

It is our duty to remain mobile and strong!

If you are planning on living into your 80's or beyond, it defines logic to stop taking care of the body you intend to use for all those years while you're still in your 40's or 50's.

Correct?

If you don't approach every day as an opportunity to move your health forward, you're doing an injustice to yourself and those around you. When your health fails, you throw a massive roadblock in front of others...not just yourself!

When we start to think of mental and physical health as a broader obligation, a greater meaning emerges.

Many people shy away from working out or vigorous movement of any kind, because they think lifting weights and running or other various forms of exercise are simply too hard or even traumatic to the body.

I suggest just the opposite.

Because we were designed as innately physical beings, when we stop behaving this way, our systems don't know how to handle it.

Disease conditions are the result.

The true trauma to our bodies is slowing down and stopping regular physical activity.

Picture a world, not too long ago, when life was relatively harsh. Simple day-to-day existence required CONSIDERABLE physical effort.

Leading a sedentary lifestyle was NOT an option.

Diabetic and pre-diabetic conditions, along with heart disease, high blood pressure and other disease states are the direct result of the traumatic effect of a sedentary lifestyle.

Leading a sedentary lifestyle is completely foreign to our physiology.

In fact, by now you may have seen or heard about the research pointing towards the significant dangers of remaining seated for long periods of time.

In a very brief period, just a few decades, we went from very active to the complete opposite. Mix in a typical "Western" diet and you have the formula for disaster.

Honestly, how could our bodies and minds NOT react poorly?

It does not take much to see the benefits of putting our body to use.

An activity as simple as walking can lengthen your lifespan. While we will spend time talking about the tremendous benefits of strength training, walking can be the gateway.

In fact, studies not only show that those who walk regularly live longer, but those who make an effort to walk at a faster pace live longer still!

Again, just doing 'stuff' we were meant to do anyway!

Our next purpose:

<u>One cannot ignore the mind-body connection.</u>

Many of us view our mindset as a separate entity from our bodies. Nothing could be further from the truth. Our way of thinking and acting when dealing with stress, as well as our relationships and community involvement, our philosophy, and our general outlook have a direct impact on our state of health.

The mind and body (our attitude and physicality, if you will) are inseparable.

We can see simple examples of this when we get sick during a particularly stressful period. Stress compromises our immune system and the result is illness. The mind and the body cannot be treated as two separate entities.

More and more studies are showing that people who have a positive outlook live longer.

This goes far beyond simple genetics and lifestyle.

This is why the Successful Aging Academy (SAA) spends so much time on "Mindset".

This is a vast topic touching upon issues such as: Goal setting, meditation, social connections, stress reduction & anxiety, motivation and much more.

The initial phase of the SAA system focuses almost exclusively on mindset.

Once you put a resilient mindset in place – anything is possible!

Without getting your mindset squared away first, making any improvements, even small ones, to any area of life can be difficult.

Conversely, there are few things in nature more powerful than a laser-focused human mind!

This leads us to our next purpose.

Nutrition.

Food can be your best friend or your most powerful enemy.

We will spend considerable time talking about nutrition. If one of your concerns is weight loss, nutrition will be approximately 65 to as much as 80% of the solution you're after.

This means you could have the greatest workout in the world, but if your nutrition is poor, you are simply spinning your wheels. You will not make progress. Food can fuel your life or it can put a halt to it.

As the expression goes, "You cannot out-train a bad diet."

Food has the power to impact virtually every system in our body, and can even turn genes on and off.

Unfortunately, much of the food we now eat comes from an industry designed solely for profit and convenience of production, rather than health. As a result, much of what we've been told about food since we were children has now been proven to be incorrect.

One of the clearest explanations for this comes for the excellent book, "In Defense of Food" by Michael Pollan. I strongly recommend adding this to your reading list, if you feel nutrition is your downfall.

As little as one century ago obesity was an anomaly, but since the mid-70s, this has all changed. Today, the majority of the population is either overweight or obese. Obesity is rampant to the point of being epidemic.

Once we have finished our coverage of food and nutrition, you will see just how simple this topic really is. You will also master the steps needed to pinpoint your nutritional trouble spots and erase them completely.

The next time you go food shopping, keep this in mind: There are entities out there that have gone out of their way to create the state of confusion regarding food today – especially in the United States.

They have managed to take something as simple and straightforward as eating, and made it wildly complicated.

False claims…

Deceptive advertising…

Questionable science…

How? As I stated earlier, when confusion exists…when making a change is confusing, people invariably revert to old habits.

They avoid making any change at all.

They choose not to choose.

We keep eating what we always have, in the same amounts, prepared the same way. Nothing changes. *Even if we consciously know something must change, because what we are doing now is not working.*

Only when the confusion is removed is positive action likely to happen.

Disrupting the status quo becomes a given!

Does any of this resonate with you yet?

I hope so.

To get a concrete view of the program that could turn things around for you...or someone you love. Please go to:

www.successfulaging.academy

The fastest, clearest way to find your starting point.

CHAPTER 3

LOSING MY SENSE OF INVINCIBILITY

I mentioned at the beginning of the book that I had a story about suddenly facing a challenge. It's one of those times where you get completely caught off guard…and shaken to the core.

Well, I actually have two such stories.

Here is the first one.

This event completely changed how I viewed myself, my health, and my entire approach to aging in general.

I pray it saves you having to go through a similar experience.

As you recall, one overriding foundation of the Successful Aging Academy is represented by our core question: "Are you ready?"

Well, in this case, I was not.

Sometimes we create a false illusion of who we are and what we are capable of doing (Expectations); refusing to acknowledge the loss of abilities due to inaction.

Well, life has a way of slapping us back to reality, sometimes in a very dramatic way. I experienced one such turn of events.

This experience moved me from the category of false illusion to one of action.

I've grown up with a very active lifestyle. From little league to collegiate All-American to a member of the US National Track and Field Team, I have always been involved with sports. I played baseball, hockey, football, etc.

To this day, I still lift weights regularly, golf, and maintain regular cardio-vascular workouts.

I also grew up around swimming pools my entire life. Like many people, I've been swimming ever since I was young and I never really thought much about it. Over the years though, this turned into more of "wading" than true swimming, and jumping off of the back of the boat for a quick dip in the lake was never an issue.

I felt comfortable around the water.

Our family is fortunate enough to have spent a good deal of time on Lake Winnesquam in New Hampshire. It is the third largest lake in New Hampshire, and is a beautiful, calm place I have come to equate with relaxation.

One of our favorite spots is a small inlet at one end of the lake called the Loon Sanctuary. Much of this section is off-limits to boaters, providing a safe breeding ground for the Loons (large relatives of ducks, if you are unfamiliar). The entire area is surrounded by trees with really only a few homes dotting the lakeside. Many times there may be only one or two boats there. As a result, it is always calm and beautifully peaceful.

One day, we were out for a boat ride and anchored in this area. It was a beautiful warm summer day. Just idyllic.

While packing up for the day, one of those inflatable 'wanna-be" life preserver "floaties" my son had been using blew overboard. I insisted he go get it, but he was all dried off and refused to go back into the water. This 'discussion' went on back and forth for a minute or so. Meanwhile, the float was drifting further and further away, pushed by the wind and the slow current of the lake.

I was getting annoyed at my son by this point, and at the thought losing the floatie, so I jumped in to go after it. In retrospect, it was a bit silly to get all annoyed. The thing could not have cost more than a dollar, but it seemed wasteful to let it go; not to mention that we would be polluting the lake with plastic.

As I was swimming towards it, it continued to drift away; a bit like a cartoon or one of those Hitchcock movies where the hallway just keeps getting longer as you reach for it...30 yards, 40 yards, 50 yards...I would stop every once in a while, saying to myself, "Where the hell is this thing?"

I was still very irritated, and also starting the get a bit fatigued.

It is important to understand a point of physics here. The total distance I swam by this point was not excessive for a regular swimmer. But...I am what you would call a 'sinker'. I can recall swimming class back at Boston University. The instructor had a technique he would show everyone on how to stay floating on water if you were in a situation similar to this.

Literally, everyone else in the class could float. I sank like a stone. This did not help my progress at the moment...

I finally reached the floatie, and realized I had covered a lot of distance. My arms and legs were alarmingly tired. There was no way I was getting back to the boat carrying this foolish $1.00 floatie, and I was too tired to climb on top of it. It was the type with a solid middle and not even little handles on the side. It was just a plastic disk. I couldn't just put my arms through and rest – not a very helpful design at the moment.

I was in a cove and I thought to myself, "I am much closer to the shore than I am to the boat. Let's go for the shoreline."

This was now a struggle. I quickly realized, without wanting to panic, things had deteriorated from a casual swim to a far more threatening situation.

My arms and legs felt like lead. Each movement required a huge effort.

Meanwhile, my children could see that I was struggling and hopped onto some more $1.00 floaties that were on the boat and started to swim over to me. Upon reflection, I'm not sure what they intended to do once they got to me. I significantly outweighed both of them...but I certainly appreciated their effort and instincts.

On this particular day, my mother, who was in her 70's, was also sitting in the boat watching all of this unfold. Although a swimmer her whole life, today she made a far better decision than I did. She knew full well she could no longer swim this distance. In reality, had she tried to, it would likely have made things worse. She correctly decided to stay in the boat.

Just to top things off, even my two dogs were there; perched on the side rail of the boat just wondering what all the commotion was about. Rescue dogs they are not. Each one weighed about ten pounds.

It really is remarkable what goes through your head in a situation like this. I thought, "This is really, really going to suck if I drown in front of my entire family here. I'm really not good at swimming anymore. I'm a 'sinker' and this was really a bad decision."

I was literally out of my depth.

By this time, I had discarded the floatie. It was only making things worse. It had to be the worst designed "floatation device" ever created. I had to try anything to get to the shore. I tried every swimming stroke possible to get there, and even inventing some new ones; anything to get to the shore.

I could hardly move my legs anymore, and could no longer lift my arms above my head.

My wife had gone onshore earlier into a little forested area with some paths and was picking blueberries. She heard the commotion and came running down to the waterside.

I was now about 20 yards from shore. It might as well have been a mile. I could hardly move.

She yelled to me "Are you OK?" I gasped back "No!" At this point, the water was maybe 8-10 feet deep, deeper than your average swimming pool with no chance of me touching the bottom.

She had to come out into the water to reach me. I was in panic mode by this point. She was able to grab onto me and eventually me get to shore. Had I been another 20 yards out, quite frankly, I'm not sure she would have succeeded.

I remember clearly reaching desperately with my feet trying to touch bottom. I thought, "Just let me touch bottom and I know I'll be OK."

Finally we reached shore. When I was able to stand on solid ground, I was wobbly and gasping for air in a way I had never experienced. The nail beds of my fingers and toes were blue.

I felt incredibly weak.

It took about 15 minutes to fully recover. My kids were all the way there by now and looking at me with a bit of shock in their eyes. It was so unexpected, everyone was caught off guard.

Once I felt able, there was only one way back. I climbed on top of that god-forsaken flotation device and swam back to the boat.

For hours, I was silent.

I didn't speak, nor did I want to. I felt a mixture of embarrassment and anger, coupled with the realization that I was no longer 'invincible'.

I had no business putting myself in that situation.

Despite my background in sports and a career in the fitness industry, I could no longer do everything I wanted to do. I was accustomed to succeeding. I could generally try something new and be pretty decent at it. I held records. I was an All-American athlete, after all!

At some point, that guy went away.

Fortunately for me, that day was not the end of my life. But, it certainly was a wake-up call.

Things had changed. I was 50 now. I wasn't invincible.

Once I had time to reflect, it also occurred to me... how many times do events like this happen every day, and the individual involved does not survive? How many lives are lost every year to sudden death, which could have easily been prevented with even a little bit of preparation?

This event, even more than my involvement with the fitness industry, prompted me to create a plan – a movement really – to help others.

In truth, I felt an obligation to do so. Both for my own future and those I can impact.

The earliest version of the Successful Aging Academy was born. I knew that if I intended to dictate my own future, I had to embrace action. Powerful change has to take place.

I was FAILING in my obligation to my family and those around me.

I was compromising my future options by making poor decisions at age 50.

Was there any reason for me to be walking about at 240 pounds – whether I lifted weights or not? Of course not!

Was I doing enough to protect my heart and brain from decay? Absolutely not!

Was the path I was on – even as a fitness professional – acceptable? NO.

And NO ONE else was going to make this change for me.

I am the one and only person who is in charge of my health!

In some form or another, this type of thing happens to people every day.

Someone realizes they can no longer jog around the block. Sprinting is out of the question. A dad discovers he really can't field a ball his son hit towards him. His range of motion simply isn't there.

A mom looks in the mirror to see an overweight physique where a lean woman used to be.

A flight or two up some stairs now seems daunting.

We may not be able to take on the same physical challenges we could when we were younger and these challenges may take longer to complete but, with some adjustments, virtually anything is possible. Any task, from weight loss to activities including climbing, running, swimming, rowing, biking, etc. is not the sole province of the young!

As we age, sometimes it is easier to sit back and let life happen to you. This is the mindset we are seeking to destroy in the Successful Aging Academy©.

Remember, inertia is evil.

It is time to be honest. If your doctor asked you why you don't take better care of yourself, what would be your response?

- "I just don't have time. Between my work, the kids, and all that, it never seems to stop."
- "I've been busting my butt for my entire life. I work/worked damn hard. I'm entitled to relax a bit."
- "I'm too old to start working out. I never have and I've been fine so far."
- "I am on the run all the time. I get plenty of exercise just doing my thing every day."
- "It hurts to exercise. My joints ache all the time."

The reasons why we start to be *observers of our own life* instead of active players can be many.

Between jobs, children, and our many daily obligations, one of the first things pushed to the bottom of the schedule is our own health and well-being. **Inertia** is now fully entrenched. We convince ourselves we are too busy, too stressed, too this or that to stay on top of things.

Starting a new process is hard.

Changing schedules is a challenge.

But it can and must be done!

The old expression "Don't reinvent the wheel" certainly applies here.

I would NOT recommend you wait for a near death experience in order to become open to change, or to come to grips with your aging and mortality.

It gets a bit frightening. Believe me.

You can, however, dive deeper into my reasons behind forming the Successful Aging Academy for someone exactly like you. Take a few minutes and find out more here:

www.successfulaging.academy

CHAPTER 4

MINDSET

When it comes to developing a strong mindset, it helps to know "why" you're looking to make a change in the first place.

Every bad habit destroyed, every new positive habit created, MUST be backed with a clear purpose. Simon Senek's book, "Start with Why" explains this concept far better than I can.

In short, it means having the courage to keep drilling down on your reasoning until you come up with the real reason you want to be a successful ager.

More often than not, it goes far beyond the "I want to tone up and lose a few pounds".

When clients would say that to me, I would stay with the "Why?" line of questioning until the true reasoning was revealed.

Here are some of the true, deeper reasons I have heard over time. You may recognize some of them, but many will be as truly unique as you are:

- I'm 50. I just got divorced, and don't want to end up alone.

- My father (or mother) died young, and I refuse to let that happen to me.

- I lost a friend my age this year. That scared me. That won't be me.

- My doctor told me to lose 30 pounds or I could easily die of a heart attack.

- The thought of me not being there for my kids keeps me up at night.

- I can feel myself losing my ability to move well and it bothers me a lot!

One of the first exercises you'll see in the Successful Aging Academy© workbook is an exercise you are required to complete: Finding your "why".

It is imperative to verbalize your driving force.

On those days when you are just a bit too tired of the fight, you will need this driving force to fall back on. Just as important, having a crystal clear focus gives you a cause to fight for…not some vague mission.

The next question we have to ask ourselves as we begin a journey back to health is this:

What's stopping me?

What is my biggest obstacle getting in the way of my successful aging plan?

When we have the answer to these question, we can destroy the rationale behind the excuses, and start to take back control.

The first phase of the Successful Aging System is based around habit change – or as the world of psychology would put it – behavioral modification.

This is how it works…

Pick one habit you want to target. (Of course, there are two ways to look at this. You may wish to break a bad habit or start a good one.)

For this example, let's focus on a bad habit you would like to break. Eating processed carbohydrates.

This is a pretty common problem for most people.

In order to keep things simple, let's group our processed carbs into what are called "the white foods"… mainly bread, rice, cereal, pasta and crackers. I realize there are plenty more examples, but bear with me…

For most people, cutting out all of these foods all at once would be next to impossible.

But, if you focus your attention on just one of them, say crackers, the task looks a lot more manageable. Keep in mind, the entire process does not have to happen overnight!

You need to commit to any habit for a long enough period of time, in order to make the mental shift from "this is something I need to do" to more of a "this is just what I do". With time, it becomes a natural part of your behavior.

How long is this timeframe? While I have heard the figure of 21 days used often, truly rewiring the brain will take longer than that. Some research indicates that 75 days may be more accurate.

Having what is called a 'replacement behavior" ready is part of this process.

In our example case, we might make statements like, "When I am looking for a snack, I always eat (blank)." Where (blank) is your new alternative. Of course, "crackers" is not allowed to be the answer! It becomes something like: mixed nuts, fruit, slices of turkey breast, etc.

Habit change is the repetition of small behaviors repeated again and again until they become engrained.

It is equally important to reward the small victories.

If crackers are a problem area for you, successfully cutting them out is a great win. You then allow yourself to enjoy that win somehow. The only rule is that the food (or habit) in question, cannot be a part of the reward.

The process might look like this:

1. **Write your "Why" statement.** You MUST pinpoint your powerful purpose of change.

2. **Form your support team.** Studies show that if you have someone to support your efforts, your success rate doubles. Therefore, you need to intentionally form a "support team" before you get started. Assume nothing here. Tell them exactly what your goal is, and ask them if they are willing to back up your efforts. Their support may come in many forms, from doing the food shopping for you – minus the crackers, to helping you identify what you will eat instead.

3. **Find your trigger(s).** That is, when does the urge to eat crackers hit you the hardest? Is it lunchtime? Is it eating crackers while watching TV in the evening? Are crackers your 'go to' mid-morning snack? Is it a combination of these scenarios?

4. **Determine ahead of time what your replacement behavior will be.** Will you change what you eat for

lunch? Will you pack something you find just as satisfying for your mid-morning snack?

5. **Break your "change" into small, achievable steps**. This will allow you to see progress, hit small but positive milestones, and to NOT be intimidated by the magnitude of a big audacious goal (B.A.G.).

6. **Stick with that one small change for a minimum of 21, but more realistically, closer to 75 days.** Going without crackers for a while is not a life changing event. However, it is one small victory over processed carbs.

You have now practiced a viable strategy, and can move onto the next food on your target list. Maybe it's rice, bread, pasta…your choice. This small victory over crackers will provide enough reinforcement for you to move forward with a confidence level you did not have a month earlier.

Now, a true habit change process can be far more elaborate than this. In fact, it could include any or all of the following:

- Goal setting
- Visualization
- Accountability coaching
- Meditation

- Stress reduction
- Self-talk
- And more...

The key point to remember: Attempting to make a massive change all at once or multiple, large changes, is a recipe for disaster!

You can and will achieve monumental change when you break the task into small, achievable goals.

Back to our example:

Goal: No more crackers

Step 1: No crackers after 8:00pm

Step 2: No crackers after 6:00pm

Step 3: No crackers at work

Step 4: No crackers during weekdays

Step 5: No crackers at social events

Step 6: etc...

As you can see, none of these steps individually are massive, but once broken down, crackers quickly become a thing of the past.

The length of these steps can vary, but it's the process of moving forward with a distinct plan that matters!

Let's take wine for example. For many people, much of their caloric intake comes from wine in the evening. I know from experience, that if a client tells me they have 1-2 glasses of wine in the evening, the truth is more like 2-4 glasses.

Let's say I asked you to drink one glass less per day than you do now...just during the weekdays.

First, let's do some math. One glass of wine contains roughly 125 calories in a 5 ounce glass. (we will ignore the fact that few people pour themselves only 5 ounces while drinking at home.)

So...here's the current scenario.

125 x 2 glasses/day = 250 calories per day...times seven days per week.

That equals 1750 calories PER WEEK. Times 52 weeks equals 91,000 calories per year!

These numbers are pretty substantial.

However, drinking even one less glass per day saves you 45,500 calories per year.

What gets tough is the old "one pound of fat contains 3,500 calories" statistic we see in articles. This figure is highly debatable. But, if we use this figure for the sake of argument, this translates to the equivalent of 13 pounds per year. Of course, there are many factors at play here, metabolically speaking.

However, the reality is that 45,500 is a reliable number, and YES, all other things being equal, you WILL lose weight by taking this one small step daily.

Success is, therefore, a habit to be practiced in small steps each day.

In summary:

Select one of your biggest obstacles, and only focus on that one thing. This is your "Big Rock". Don't attempt to make any other wholesale changes to your diet right now.

Grab that success and make a game out of breaking the next poor habit – or creating the next good habit.

Other Mindset Issues:

On being 'resilient'

Resilience refers to the ability bounce back from a challenge or adversity. As we age, clearly we face more challenges and adversity. It's just how life goes...

Those of us over 45 or 50 often find ourselves in a position to be the 'rock' of our family unit. Life does not ask us whether or not we are ready for this title.

Isn't it, therefore, our responsibility to be resilient?

If 'resilient' is NOT the first thing people think of when your name is mentioned, not to worry. This is a trait that can be learned.

Developing a resilient mindset is another core tenet of the Successful Aging Academy©. Without it, each issue life throws at us can throw us into a tailspin. If that happens often enough, and we fail to recover, we become of little help to those around us…or to ourselves.

Each of us should come to view resilience as a requirement, a duty. Master it with constant practice.

Accountability

You may think that successful people, those at the top of their game, just have a certain gift. Maybe they're just a little smarter, have more will power, were dealt a better hand…all that.

Not true.

Some of the most well-known 'overachievers' have been very purposeful when it comes to surrounding themselves with people who hold them accountable.

Yes, they dream big, but they have others in their lives who will hold them accountable for completing each step required to achieve those dreams.

Accountability is key.

If you don't have deadlines and/or expectations to meet, tasks – even important ones – can drift.

Let's say you have a family vacation scheduled, but have a huge work-related (or home-related) project that MUST be completed prior to your departure? I think we can all identify with this.

Aren't you astounded to see exactly how much you can get accomplished in the days prior to your leaving? You become laser focused on the task at hand and allow nothing to get in your way!

Well, having someone to hold you accountable is pretty much like that.

They will not let you drift. They know what your goals are and will call you out if you don't stay the course!

Being open to having someone as your accountability partner is step one.

However, holding ourselves accountable is far more challenging. If you have a system in place, you have a greater chance of success, but for the average person, holding yourself accountable is a skill that must be refined over years of practice.

Accountability is at the core of the Successful Aging Academy© system. Fortunately, we live in a time where we can use technology to help us fight the battle.

A Mindset Side Note

I think we're all familiar with the 'victim' mentality.

This occurs when someone insists their lack of success, or the reason behind their negative actions or habits can be blamed on someone or something else. They are not personally to blame.

They are simply a victim.

All personal responsibility is absent.

This mentality takes all the pressure off the individual. The ability to blame others for all the bad things in our lives takes us off the hook. We can coast along living under the delusion that we are victims of a great conspiracy.

I have seen a very dangerous twist on this theme in the area of health and fitness.

Using similar psychology, many people who have let themselves go have adapted the mentality of "I'm OK with how I look", or "I am comfortable with my body and who I am."

While it is important to have a positive self-image, taking this mentality too far is dangerous.

I am referring to individuals who allow themselves to become extremely overweight, and only then adopt the approach of "I'm comfortable with my size."

Being comfortable with one's size does NOT prevent disease.

Accepting one's body for what it is will not halt the progress of diabetes, heart disease, high blood pressure and early death. Like the victim mentality, taking this approach removes the discomfort required to lose weight in order to live a more healthy lifestyle.

I fully realize this may not be a politically popular position these days. But seldom is the entire picture presented showing the impact of someone's early death upon other family members left behind.

The medical costs of a lifetime of diabetes medication and treatment will not be lessened because someone is 'comfortable with their size'.

Before you start writing letters and sending emails chastising me about my callousness towards issues of self-image and confidence, understand that I am all for these things.

Having a positive self-image is a prerequisite for a happy, fulfilling life.

However…

I'm simply stating that the real health issues associated with obesity remain unchanged by popular psychology.

The victim mentality has no place at SAA.

If I eat too much – my fault.

If I drink too much – that's on me.

If I blow off the gym – my decision.

Never let the 'blame game' become a part of your thought process.

Let's be clear, the next step after becoming a victim is becoming a slave... a slave to your own poor health... trapped in a body that no longer functions as it should.

Instead of this "I'm OK with the way I am" mentality, ask yourself this question, "What can I do so this never happens to me again?"

"What steps can I take to be the owner of my health and longevity again?"

Like the mantra says, "I dictate my own future". That starts with taking ownership of your decision-making process, not participating in the blame game and never passing the buck.

The "Disruptor" Mindset and the Power of Change

I spend a lot of time talking about disruption. I believe it is such an important concept that I want to make EVERYONE over age 45 a disruptor! This is definitely a new way of looking at your daily decisions and even your life in general; so the concept deserves another mention.

Elon Musk is a disruptor. From Telsa to Space X, he comes at things from different angles, and usually ends up changing entire industries. The creators of Uber revolutionized the taxi industry by changing the status quo.

<u>A Disruptor is anyone who refuses to accept the current version of 'normal'.</u>

You may or may not change the world the way Elon Musk did, but you can certainly disrupt your own world to a significant degree.

Here's how…

Take one personal pattern, something you have been doing a certain way for as long as you can remember, and starting today, do it differently.

Here are some examples:

- Use Stevia instead of sugar in your coffee
- Take one more flight of stairs per day than you currently do
- If you ALWAYS use a 15 pound dumbbell for a certain exercise, try the 20's for at least the first set
- If you always stay up to watch a certain program, during the week, try recording it and going to bed ½ hour earlier.
- Go one week without your normal dessert
- If you drink alcohol, change the pace at which you drink to a slower one. Most people I know have been conditioned to drink at a certain pace. Slow it down and alternate with sips with water.

- Grill, roast, or steam one new veggie recipe. Learning a new way to prepare food is a great way to shake things up
- Buy a larger water bottle or cup and keep it full of water on your desk or table
- Pick a different time of day to workout. A time that normally might be wasted time.

You get the point. These are not exactly earth-shaking changes, but this is how healthy disruptions start.

Pick one action you have NEVER done before, and add it to your routine…and I chose the word "routine" carefully.

Routine can be the enemy!

"If you always do as you always have, you will always get what you always got."

For many people, myself included, routines are not always good. So what do I plan on changing up? Recently, I started working out before my workday starts. Once I got into the habit, I found I got more done during the day, since I did not have to worry about getting my workout done later. I also noticed I had significantly more energy throughout the day, because I fired up my nervous system early.

I simply took a time of day that was otherwise unproductive and moved something important there. I completely disrupted my daily pattern, and saw very positive results.

A little different…and a change from my regular patterns. Keep in mind, I have been working out for over 40 years, but NEVER did I train in the early morning.

Now, I couldn't imagine doing it at any other time of day.

Disrupting your life in some way can be a scary thing. Many of us have made decisions that changed the course of our lives. Such decisions have had a huge impact on my life.

The decision to alter my own training to include more cardio-vascular training, as well as swimming more often, was a direct result of my near-drowning incident. It took that level of drama to move me to action.

As a professional in the fitness industry, I have spent my entire life urging people to change, trying to motivate and inspire people to take control of their lives and their health in any way I can.

One of the single most difficult things to do is to create a change in someone's behavior. In my industry, knowing how to do this is THE key to success, and one of the cornerstones of the entire profession.

While I have had significant success helping people make healthy changes and achieve their goals, there are some who failed to do so. I failed to get through to them.

I couldn't come up with that one trigger that clicked with them.

So why is persuading someone to change so difficult?

I see two key parts to this answer:

It all comes back to routines. Rote behavior if you will.

There is a cue, a routine we follow as a result of this cue, and then a reward. Humans find comfort in routine. This routine can become deeply engrained in our everyday behavior. Convincing someone to disrupt their routine is a monumental task.

Consider this.

Most of us eat pretty much the same food, prepared the same way, and in the same amount, pretty much all the time.

Variation is the exception, not the rule.

For example, to a cigarette smoker, lighting up a cigarette in the morning while grabbing a cup of coffee can be part of a highly engrained morning routine. Not only does the smoker have a physical need to bring his or her nicotine levels back up, but this rote behavior is part of a ritual…part of who they are.

This explains why quitting is so difficult.

It goes well beyond the addictive properties of the cigarette itself.

Next, if I am going to persuade you to abandon your routine, and go down a completely different path, there needs to be – at its core – some deeply powerful emotion.

This is the "Why" exercise we discussed earlier.

Our deeply engrained, rote behaviors can only be broken when we are ready to disrupt our thought patterns, based upon a powerful trigger or "Why".

If you have yet to write down the nature of your "Why", I implore you to do it before you go on.

If you have tried and failed to make permanent, lasting change, it doesn't mean you have failed.

It proves you had the wrong system in place. You chose the incorrect vehicle. Nothing more.

The power of your mind is vast beyond understanding. And to be clear, when it is harnessed to serve you and your goals, you become virtually unstoppable.

Once you have this clarity...once you put the right system in place, you will look back at those past failures as little more than speedbumps.

Make these blips on your road to inevitable success and the rediscover of the best version of you.

The first step is presented here:

www.successfulaging.academy

CHAPTER 5

ADDITIONAL MENTAL AND PHYSICAL CONSIDERATIONS

Let's state this up front.

It is quite possible that few things we encounter daily can kill you as quickly as stress.

The thing is, we need stress to live. It's been said that the only people who have no stress are dead. I believe this.

It's stress in excess where the trouble starts.

Here is a list – not definitive by any means, of the things we KNOW stress does to our bodies.

<u>Your body:</u>

Headache, chest pain, high blood pressure, pounding heart, clenching jaws, sleep issues, weight gain/loss, fatigue, diarrhea, shortness of breath, upset stomach

Internally, you can experience feelings of:

Anxiety, worrying, irritability, forgetfulness, mood swings, sadness, poor concentration, negativity, anger, depression, insecurity and burn out

All of this can result in behaviors that include:

Loss of appetite, outbursts of anger, social isolation, decreased job performance, abuse of recreational drugs and alcohol, conflicts with family and friends

Many of us have become so used to experiencing stress on a daily basis that we consider it standard operating procedure. But, this is far from normal.

We simply are not designed to experience chronic stress on a daily basis.

There are two major types of stress; chronic and acute. Stress can also be emotional and physical. Let's stick with emotional for now. Also, for this discussion I will be ignoring eustress (good stress) since that is not usually a concern with regard to a negative health impact.

Here's the difference. Acute stress is a one-time event. Face a crisis. Execute the fight or flight response. Crisis over.

Chronic stress is entirely different, and a rather new phenomenon. Being the brilliant humans we are, we have figured out a way to be stressed all the time.

We can experience chronic stress day in and day out for years.

This type of stress relies largely upon cortisol. There are also some other chemicals at work here, but let's focus on this one for now.

An example of how cortisol works in our daily life is when you wake up in the morning about 5 minutes before your alarm goes off. Cortisol is what woke you up.

This is useful stuff. It keeps you at a level of arousal and alertness throughout your day. Cortisol is also supposed to follow normal cycles throughout the day. Elevating in the morning to wake you up and then decreasing at night so you can sleep.

However, the pressures of our work and family life, as well as many lifestyle choices, can throw these cycles out of whack.

The result is sleep disruption, and a subsequent cascade of health problems as listed above.

In fact, stress has been shown in studies to actually age the brain more quickly by 'remodeling' and shrinking the brain. It may also be a catalyst for brain diseases such as Alzheimer's Disease and dementia.

You may say, "I don't have control over these stress levels." And this may be true. The sources of your stress may be job or family related, and truly may be beyond your control.

If this it truly the case, it is your obligation to seek healthy ways to deal with this stress.

The most common ways of doing so are through tools such as meditation or mindfulness-based stress reduction and exercise.

These options are much more readily available than they used to be. I strongly encourage you to search out such solutions. The consequences are too severe to let this slide.

"Fix Sleep First"

This leads nicely to our next topic.

If you're anything like me, you can name on one hand the number of people you know who DON'T have sleep issues.

A good night's sleep goes far beyond determining your energy levels. In fact, the impact on your physical and mental health is far-reaching, and perhaps even more important than any other pattern in your life.

Sound dramatic? It should.

My experience with clients has been that if someone is having trouble losing weight, getting to the gym, eating poorly, etc., once we take a close look at their sleep patterns and target the trouble spots there, many of the other pieces fall into place.

I tell clients and audiences the same thing, "Fix sleep first!" This will absolutely be the best 'bang for your buck' when it comes to energy levels, as well as mental and physical well-being.

In fact, a recent study showed a previously unknown process that occurs in the human brain. It seems that during sleep, the brain essentially "cleans out" waste products much like a street sweeper cleaning the empty streets at night.

However, this system ONLY functions properly during extended, uninterrupted hours of sleep. It effectively shuts down when sleep is disturbed.

Here is just a partial list of the areas that can impact sleep:

- Nutritional status
- Supplement status

- Physical activity
- Stress levels
- Work hours and responsibilities
- Relationship status
- Sleeping environment & distractions
- Even pets

Here's the thing. If you look at the above list, you will see that almost all of these are under your control. It is key for each of us to examine our own sleep patterns, identify disruptions that may exist, and fix them at all costs.

Proper sleep will then positively influence every other aspect of our lives from how we handle stress, how resilient we are with challenges, our creativity levels, job performance, dietary choices, relationships, and on and on…

Exercise: If a full, deep and restful night's sleep is rare for you, you have a responsibility to determine the reasons why and correct them!

Community, social networks and relationships

Talk about a huge topic!

Obviously, entire books are written on any of these. However, they are being mentioned here solely for their impact on longevity.

It has been proven time and time again that if you have a strong sense of community, participate in thriving social networks, and make efforts to build strong interpersonal relationships, your quality of life and length of life will improve.

There are several reasons why individuals can lose one or all of these benefits.

Death of family and friends could leave you alone.

A loss of independence and mobility could physically limit your access to these groups.

An increasing sense of self-imposed isolation can also be a factor.

However, this is one area where stepping out of your comfort zone can have tremendous positive impact.

It can be easy for some of us to fall into a more isolated existence; especially given the ease of internet access to a wealth of information and entertainment.

However, humans are naturally highly social animals, and need face-to-face interaction with others. This keeps our brain stimulated and our social skills sharp.

In fact, stated flatly, I believe it is virtually impossible to age successfully without a strong sense of community and reliable long-lasting relationships.

We have created a reference library, of sorts, at the Successful Aging Academy.

Looking for a Stress Reduction action plan? Done.

In need of a detailed plan to fix your sleep issues? It's here.

Is nutrition your downfall? We have built a step by step plan to remove the lies and myths.

We're now going to jump into the fitness piece of the Academy. If you need a starting point, you'll find it here as well.

www.successfulaging.academy

CHAPTER 6

WORKOUT DESIGN 101

The Story of the 10 Pound Woman

I'll never forget this client. Her name was Joanne. While Joanne was somewhat active and an avid golfer, she maintained a belief she was much older and less capable than she truly was. I mean FAR less capable. She was actually only 64 at the time. This may have been older than my average client, but certainly not as old as she perceived herself to be.

Joanne had convinced herself she could only use the very lightest dumbbells for the majority of her exercises, even when it was clear she could lift far more. Bear in mind, she was a bit stubborn, and was convinced she was correct about her presumptions. This attitude served her well in other aspects of her life; but in this situation, it was a clear handicap.

Quite often, when I handed her a pair of ten pound dumbbells, she would look at me with surprise in her eyes and ask, "Are you sure this isn't too much"? I replied, "I'm very sure. Give it a try." Of course, she was able to complete the set quite easily. You can imagine the looks I received when I handed her the fifteen pound dumbbells!

Joanne's golf game magically improved. Often, I told her the dumbbells were a certain weight, and I suspected she knew the truth; but I often tricked her into challenging herself. She looked better and felt better. It was just like magic.

How does this mindset come about?

How does an otherwise healthy individual convince him or herself they are weak to the point of disability, yet the only 'condition' present is being chronologically older than a certain percentage of the population?

Are there any situations where you put similar limitations on yourself?

The alarming part of the story is that it is not so unique. Many older adults are convinced they are incapable of doing certain tasks. I don't mean you should go to the gym today and try to deadlift 400 pounds just because some younger gym member can do it. But…you MUST start somewhere.

In short, once you stop moving – due to either age or occupation – a downward spiral of health is virtually certain.

Most people view this downward spiral as a natural consequence of aging, when in fact it is a consequence of lifestyle choice.

Here's the irony: just when we reach the point where our body begins to show its age by reducing hormone production and losing muscle mass; just when we need activity the most to prevent and fight the signs of aging, most adults stop moving altogether!

This is completely contradictory to what we should be doing.

When exercise becomes a necessity for survival, most of us stop doing it.

Which came first? Did we grow old because we stopped moving, or did we stop moving because we perceive ourselves as old?

Recently, I did a presentation for the Senior Center in my home town. Most of the folks in the audience were over 60 years of age. The talk was on gluten and grains, but inevitably the conversation touched upon strength training.

When I stated EVERYONE should be lifting weights, I got many stunned looks.

It was as if strength training was reserved only for the young or the occasional "fitness nut".

Strength training (also known as resistance training) is the ONLY way to preserve valuable muscle mass. One woman asked me, "How many days per week do I need to lift weights?" I am sure she was hoping I would say only one or two. I answered, "Three days per week. Minimum." She was aghast.

Many people in the room were regular walkers, which was AWESOME! People who walk regularly live longer. Period. However, walking only addresses general fitness issues. Walking will NOT preserve muscle mass, especially in the upper body. Cardio-vascular activity is vital, things like running outdoors and jogging on the treadmill, but this is only part of the health and wellness equation.

Another gentleman asked why he was actually losing weight each year. He did not want to lose weight and rightly so. He appeared to have a normal, healthy bodyweight. I commended him for his awareness of physical changes. I explained it was likely he was suffering from muscular atrophy. He was losing actual muscle tissue.

Each year after age 40 we lose up to one-half pound of muscle mass. There are many reasons why this happens, but one of the newest studies from the UK indicates that we start to lose muscle mass not just because we tend to train less as we age, but the nerves to the muscle itself can actually die off.

This is not a pleasant thought!

However, the good news is that the study also shows that people who maintain healthy muscle mass through regular strength training can prevent much of this 'natural' muscle mass loss.

NOTE: We don't have room here to list out actual programs. But, we have provided you with plenty of appropriately designed strength training programs inside SAA.

However, there are some clear concepts you should understand.

Lifting weight is what we were meant to do. We are ALL capable of lifting much more than we believe we are. Increases in strength levels can be achieved into our nineties. Fact.

In addition, resistance training (lifting weights) has been shown to have an anti-aging effect on the brain. Good enough reason for me to keep going to the weight room.

I would rather suffer through the occasional stress and strain of sore or even painful muscles, than the indignity of disabling muscular atrophy brought about by sheer inactivity.

I would go as far as to say that each of us has an *obligation* to do weight training – especially given evidence that failing to do so results in both mental and physical deterioration.

People have bought into this myth that they are too old to exercise. They should slow down and sit in a rocking chair...and wait for what?

Start slowly.

Steadily increase the frequency and volume of the load you are lifting.

Change the exercises you are doing every month or so. You must challenge the muscles or they will not grow.

Recommendation:

Lift weights for 30 minutes and then do cardio interval training for 30 minutes. Lift weights first! It is a common mistake for people to do their cardio-vascular exercise first as a way to 'warm up' and then lift weights. Unfortunately, this is the opposite of what you should be doing, since the cardio work will interfere with muscle growth. Remember it this way: whatever is done first, gets the best results.

Do strength training a minimum of 3 days per week.

Add a long *power* walk on the weekend – preferably outdoors.

Society has certain expectations for those over 50 or 60 years of age. We should all strive to DEFY these expectations. We are all capable of more.

Defy the inertia. Disrupt the status quo…on a daily basis.

Grab a heavier set of dumbbells.

We are capable of so much more.

Remember the first line of our new mantra: "I am mobile and strong."

Putting together your own workouts

Keep in mind, the purpose of this chapter, and an overriding theme to this entire book, is to provide the average person with a starting point.

How do you construct a proper workout?

First we need to establish EXACTLY what your goal is. **For our population – the over 50 crowd – muscle mass retention should be the number one priority**.

There are some experts who would disagree. They may say the focus should be on balance, mobility, flexibility or some other trait. However, with a higher degree of muscle mass comes a higher degree of functionality; nor are all these other goals mutually exclusive.

Much like sleep can be the foundation upon which many other traits are based, more muscle mass allows all the other traits listed above to prosper.

The only proven way to combat muscle mass loss is through resistance training. That's it. Yoga won't do it. Pilates won't do it, nor will distance running. While these activities have their own unique benefits, they do not increase muscle mass, which is the basis of our discussion here.

One view of the definition of health requires one to be able to complete daily tasks safely, and still be able to deal with an occasional "emergency" or physically challenging event.

For those not entirely comfortable in the gym or with resistance training in general, **here are some basic rules for your workouts:**

- Never start lifting weights until you have a light sweat going.

- Always start with light weights and work up to your target weights.

- If a particular exercise causes pain, stop immediately and switch this movement for one that does not cause pain. There is always another option. Pain is a valuable signal. Listen to it.

- Workouts should follow this sequence: dynamic warm up, strength training, cardio-vascular training, cool down, and finish with stretching. Never do cardio-vascular work before strength training.

- Know your limitations. Never let your ego get the better of you. Little is accomplished by attempting maximum effort weights over age 50.

- Strive to increase the amount of weight you use each training session; even by just a tiny bit. This could mean increasing the number of reps, increasing the weight used or increasing the number of sets completed. Using the same load for weeks, months, or even years on end will result in minimal gains, and will invariably result in stagnation and boredom.

This book is all about getting started, right? Well, in doing the research for this book, I heard a very consistent theme.

Many adults don't know how to LITERALLY get started.

I'm referring to step one of your workouts…a simple warmup.

Let's address that issue right here.

First, let's explain why we need a 'warmup' in the first place. It may seem obvious, but has anyone ever really explained the purpose?

A warmup does several things:

- It fires up the nervous system
- It increases overall blood flow
- It increases the range of motion for the muscles you are about to use
- It raises your core body temperature
- It decreases your risk of injury

All of these are vital for safe and effective workouts.

Here is your basic warmup: A proper warmup should not take any longer than 8-10 minutes maximum. In extremely cold areas, it may take a bit longer to get the blood flowing…but not much.

You may want to go through sections 3 and 4 two times each.

NOTE: A complete video demonstration of this warmup is included in the training portion of the SAA training section.

Section 1: Walk on the treadmill for 5 minutes. Use a brisk pace suitable for you. I use 3.0 mph.

Section 2: Foam roller work

- Back
- Quadiceps
- Hips

Section 3: Joint and Range of Motion work

- Arm circles
- Calf stretch
- Pec stretch against the wall
- Shoulder / Triceps stretch
- Back/Lat stretch with overhead handle
- Glute stretch

- Hip flexor stretch
- Hip rotator stretch

Section 4: Dynamic Movements

- Leg swings
- Leg grab
- Air squats
- Dynamic lunges with twists
- Lying crossovers (face up)
- Lying crossovers (face down)

The next step in a proper program design is to incorporate the following six variables.

The goal here is not be make you a strength coach, but to give you a basic understanding of resistance training. Every workout is made up of the follow pieces.

- Which specific exercises are used
- The number of sets completed
- The number of repetitions you complete in each set
- The length of the rest period between sets
- The speed or 'tempo' used to move the weight for each repetition
- How much actual weight is used for each exercise

This may look like a lot. The above list can be overwhelming since the in-depth knowledge of all this is usually left to fitness professionals.

Here's the reality. <u>You don't have to know all of the variables above.</u>

The workouts provided through the Successful Aging Academy© system handles each variable for you. You just need to look at the video on your phone when you're at the gym and follow along.

Mobility and the lack thereof...

One of the more noticeable losses that can come with age is a loss of mobility. This is not the same as flexibility. Think of mobility as being a measure of how well your entire body works together as a whole.

In daily life, an example might be having to squat down to duck under something, or the need to climb up and over something. Having to lift your leg up and over something can be a challenge, especially if you don't do anything like that on a regular basis.

Earlier in this book, we mentioned that the average person doesn't do much during a typical week that could be classified as 'athletic'. Climbing a set of stairs may be the extent of it.

By not asking the body to be mobile, mobility will be lost.

This can be a huge limiting factor in quality of life, limit certain activities, and lead to injury.

I interviewed Functional Aging Institute (FAI) founder Dan Ritchie, and discussed this very topic. One important action he recommended was to focus on the hip joint for mobility work.

He said a loss of mobility in the hips can have wide ranging negative impact. From sitting, to climbing stairs, to reaching across the body, or lunging and bending over to the ground, the movement through the hips and torso is vital.

For this reason, mobility based movements should be included in the routines of anyone over age 45. The composition of mobility circuits can be found at www.successfulaging.academy, along with complete top to bottom workouts, the warmup presented above and a complete listing of cardio-vascular workouts.

CHAPTER 7

NUTRITION

"Let food be thy medicine and medicine be thy food"

- Hippocrates

A client came to me and asked if I would be willing to work with her daughter. Her daughter was in college. I knew her daughter, since I had actually trained her when she was a younger athlete. The mom was quite concerned because her daughter had gained a large amount of weight over the past several years, and it was becoming a serious health situation.

Of course, I said I would be happy to help.

When my client came to gym the next time, I was hopeful we could schedule a time for her daughter to come in and meet with me. Unfortunately, it was not to be. Her daughter explained to her, "I can't do it. The first thing he will want me to do is to stop eating sugar, and there is no way I can do that."

Such is the addictive power of sugar.

Have no doubt about this! Sugar is *the* source of the vast majority of this country's obesity epidemic.

But honestly, sugar is just one in a long list of hurdles, delusions and fallacies many of us live with every day.

If there was ever a topic with more confusion, misinformation, and even outright lies, it's the topic of nutrition.

It is easy to become confused about what works and what does not. It seems each week a new book comes out promoting some new diet promising to help you shed pounds with ease.

Atkins, The Zone, South Beach, The Raw Diet, various forms of fasting…the options go on and on.

Adding to the confusion is the fact that much of what we – meaning anyone growing up in the 60's and 70's – have been told about nutrition is a lie! We were always told that carbohydrates are good and all fats are bad. In fact, I had a professor in college who had a coffee mug which read; "I never met a carbohydrate I didn't like".

My, how things have changed! While carbohydrates are vital for life, an excess of them in the diet inevitably leads to unhealthy weight gain.

We were also told that breads and grains are great for us. This is clearly turning out to not be the case. Eating lots of breads, even whole wheat breads, adds a huge amount high-glycemic calories to your diet, and can cause strong negative reactions to many who eat them.

"Good fats" are now emerging as a valuable nutrient with many health benefits. All fats are not bad.

All this confusion leads many people to give up. Another form of 'paralysis by analysis'.

It is important to note many nutritional approaches do work.

However, if there was only one perfect diet, we would all be on it, and obesity would not exist. Alas, life is more complicated than that.

Nutrition as a tool is SO powerful, it is going to be central to your "Ideal Me Project" planning.

You MUST be ready to disrupt what you consider to be a normal diet and be open to other options. The HC45 system will work…but only if you are willing to work with the system!

As you read this, I'm guessing it is easy for some of you to pinpoint your "Big Rock".

What is it? What is this single biggest hurdle holding you back?

Let's write it down. Break it down. Create the plan. Destroy the Big Rock.

Wishful thinking is NOT a plan!

When you do select a diet, you are at least putting some form of plan in place.

This is a great start.

Take action. Evaluate some approaches to eating and get started!

Embracing action is the first step.

That being said, I have never read a study that indicates the "Mediterranean Diet" does not improve almost all measures of health. I am a strong believer in this approach. It is really just that; an approach rather than a diet. It is a way of eating for a lifetime.

If I were to make a modification to the Mediterranean Diet, it would be to decrease the amount of grains used. Keep in mind, the population that this particular diet is based upon, were a very physical people.

Today, we are generally far less active.

Getting into detailed specifics about the Mediterranean Diet goes beyond the scope of this book. However, volumes of information are readily available regarding how to use this strategy for long-term health and weight management. Here is a very brief summary:

The Mediterranean diet emphasizes eating foods like fish, poultry, fruits, vegetables, beans, high-fiber breads and whole grains, nuts, and olive oil. Other meat, cheese, and sweets are very limited. The recommended foods are rich with monounsaturated fats, fiber, and omega-3 fatty acids.

One of the very reasons I decided to become a Certified Nutritionist was the realization that roughly 65-70% of my client's positive results were attributed to a sound nutritional approach. You can follow the greatest workouts routine ever devised, but if you don't mesh these workouts with a healthy diet, it is all for naught.

I am going to present a series of rules, followed by some straightforward rationale.

If you follow these rules, your likelihood of success in reaching your goals will increase dramatically. Remember, there is no single 'ideal' diet, or we would all be following it. Everyone has different tastes, varied daily routines and very unique metabolisms. Finding a program that works for you and more importantly, one that fits your lifestyle is the challenge.

The Rules for Nutritional Success

1) **Avoid processed foods:** These are defined as bread, white rice, cereals, pasta, crackers, pastries, and of course, all refined sugar products. The latter is generally found in the form of cookies, candies, soda, and any other sweets.

   I realize this is much easier said than done.

   For many people, the above list makes up a large portion of their diet; especially when it comes to bread.

   In addition, refined sugars have made their way into foods we used to consider healthy alternatives. Being a good label reader is vital in the battle against processed foods.

   The more man puts his hands on a food product, the worse it is for you. You can refer back to the cliché regarding the layout of the grocery store to better remember this. If it comes in a bag or a can or if the list of ingredients contains a paragraph of chemical names which you can barely pronounce, you may want to rethink it.

2) **Always have emergency foods in the house**: _In my experience this is the number one reason the majority of people fail with their nutritional plans._ If you have gone any extensive period without food, and your blood sugar is very low, you will eat whatever options are available. This is when bad choices are very often made.

Failure here is avoided by planning ahead with regular shopping for fresh foods and meal preparation. Simple things like having healthy snacks at arm's reach can prevent a significant lapse.

I recommend picking two days per week and set aside time to grill meats and steam or grill vegetables. The veggies stay good for a shorter period of time, so you may have to prepare them more frequently.

Here is a list of good emergency foods to have on hand: mixed nuts – especially cashews, walnuts, almonds, and pecans; quality sliced meats – not cured meats such as pepperoni and salami. This means good meats such as sliced turkey and chicken. Fresh fruits – especially fruits in the berry family; fresh veggies with dip; <u>natural</u> peanut butter – remember, there is NO logical reason for sugar to be an ingredient in peanut butter!

3) **If weight management is your goal, avoid dairy and grains**: This one really gets attention. In fact, I have

had debates with many who are adamant that bread has been a staple in the human diet for centuries, and cannot possibly be bad.

While largely true, it is a truth from a different time. There was an era when humans had to physically struggle on a daily basis in order to survive. A calorie dense food was vital. Bread served that purpose. Today, we do not fight the same physical battles in order to survive.

Bread should be considered a tasty treat on par with desserts, not a daily necessity.

I have seen the removal of grains for weight management work too well to ignore. Dairy also falls into this category. If you cut out dairy, you will see almost immediate progress. This includes yogurt. While I am a strong fan of cheeses of all kinds, if I need to get lean, I drop the cheese. The results will speak for themselves.

NOTE: Dropping a calorie rich food like bread is NOT appropriate for the individual who already has a reduced caloric intake due to some form of infirmity, disease condition, or advanced aging. Breads and grains may be the only way to maintain a vital intake of calories for this population. The above rule applies ONLY to individuals battling issues with excess body weight.

4) Follow the concept of 'nutrient timing': It may sound fancy, but this simply means timing your food intake with your physical activity. If you are going to the gym or doing some other form of physical exercise, time your carbohydrate intake to follow that activity within 60-90 minutes. If you must have a high sugar/carbohydrate food, this one hour window is the time to do it.

When you do this, the carbohydrates you take in are – for the most part – used to replace the energy stored in your muscles, and not stored as fat.

If you are *not* working out at all on a particular day, it is important to be mindful of how much food you are eating. In short, food high in calories should be eaten only on days when you are expending lots of calories through exercise.

Studies have shown that two individuals can be fed the exact same diet in every way, but if one person times their caloric intake properly, the weight loss difference between the two can be substantial.

A second recommendation would be to ingest the highest volume of carbohydrates at the earliest point in the day; say before noon.

5) Stay hydrated: This advice has been promoted everywhere because it is 100% true. There is no easier way to promote recovery from workouts, proper digestion, better sleep, healthier skin, and even weight loss than having adequate water intake. How much? You should strive to take in 50% of your body weight (pounds) in ounces of water every day.

I regularly keep an oversized water container with me in the house and while I drive every day. Out of habit now, I sip water every few minutes. Throughout the course of the day, I probably refill this large 24 ounce cup multiple times – maybe 4-5 times.

That's a LOT of water. I don't mind an extra trip or two to the rest room, if it keeps me well hydrated.

Remember the distance runner's advice: By the time you realize you're thirsty, it's too late. You are dehydrated.

6) **Beware of portion sizes:** While not uniquely an American issue, it certainly may have started here in the land of abundance. The rules are simple. A portion size of meat equals the size of your palm. A cup of veggies is the size of your fist. These rules are seldom followed.

There is a restaurant near my home renowned for its heaping portion sizes. They truly believe they are providing great value to their customers by heaping piles of pasta and meat onto their plate.

However, the last time we ate at this particular restaurant, my daughter, who was about five years old at the time, looked around and commented, "Dad, everyone in here is really big."

Case closed.

Portion size is not a matter of value for the dollar, it a matter of health.

7) **Write things down**. If you ever reach a plateau in your progress, starting a food log or journal will quickly change things. The very action of writing things down will make you more 'mindful' of the choices you are making. You will be less inclined to overindulge if you know you must write things down and – better yet – have this journal reviewed weekly by someone.

There are some excellent apps available which make food journaling quick and easy to do.

What do I mean by 'mindful'? Many people follow a routine when it comes to eating. They ingest food almost on a rote, automatic basis with no consideration about the actual content. If you are mindful about your choices, this means you consider the food, its content, its impact on your health, and whether or not it will move you towards or away from your goals. You should consider the amount you are consuming when you are consuming it, as well as the quality, etc.

If you implement these recommendations, you will make better choices and feel better about yourself.

The other important point about keeping a food journal is to avoid relying on "recall". Be consistent about when you write things down. There is a tendency to underestimate food consumption by up to 20% when trying to think back several days about what you actually ate; if you can remember the food content at all.

8) **Veggies, veggies, veggies:** If you got every nutritionist in the world together in a room, you would hear a lot of varied opinions on the way we should eat. However, the one thing they would likely all agree on is vegetable intake.

In short, 'the more the better' when it comes to veggies. You cannot go wrong by increasing your veggie intake. Of course, this assumes you are not deep frying them!

I have met with many clients who say, "I really don't like vegetables." My reply? "Get over it!" An aversion to veggies is usually left over from childhood when sugar was the thing that tasted good and veggies were seen as the enemy. Hopefully, our taste buds have matured since then.

In addition, veggies can be prepared in quite a variety of ways to make their taste more appealing to those who have a problem with them.

I always tell clients reluctant to eat veggies, "There are few things a little extra virgin olive oil and garlic cannot make taste good."

Again, if you can follow these rules for 80-90% of the time, you will see progress. You do not have to be a fanatic about rules, counting calories and in a constant state of deprivation, to make progress with your nutrition.

However, if your diet strays dramatically from the above rules, you may wish to reconsider some things.

What is "The Fat Gap"?

If you are anything like millions of folks out there who are struggling with a slow, steady weight gain over time, I want to propose an explanation.

Something I call "The Fat Gap".

The fat gap emerges when you eat the same foods, slowly decrease physical activity over many years, even keep your body weight consistent, and still manage to get heavier.

Having counseled hundreds of clients over the years, a certain pattern starts to emerge...especially over the age of 50.

It just doesn't seem fair.

Your body fat can increase even though you strive to maintain the same healthy patterns over time.

So how does that work? Well, a very particular set of circumstances is at work here.

Condition #1. As a general rule, people do not change their eating habits very much. While you may mix things up temporarily while on a diet, most of us stick with the same or similar foods, and usually in the same portion sizes over time.

Condition #2. Another harsh reality in life is that no matter how hard we try, our metabolism will slow as we get older. Sadly, there is not a whole lot we can do about this one. Yes, interval training and weight lifting can influence our metabolism, but the trend over time is towards a slower metabolism.

Condition #3. The next piece of the puzzle is muscle mass. While there are some exceptions, the vast majority of people lose muscle mass over time. As we become less active, we atrophy.

Additionally, one new study proved that the nerves that tell a muscle to fire actually start dying off. Without a nerve telling a muscle to fire…it just gets smaller.

The real problem with the loss of muscle mass is the equal loss of the ability to burn sugar.

Your muscles use and store large amounts of sugar (carbs) every day. Therefore, when you lose muscle mass, you lose the ability to burn as much sugar and your capacity to store it goes down as well. Yet, as we mentioned, you continue to eat the same amount of carbohydrates over time.

Even if you remain relatively active, your muscle mass will drop over time. The average person can lose up to half a pound of muscle mass per year!

The ONLY way to slow the loss of muscle mass is through strength training. Period.

You may be able to see where I am headed with this. When you combine Condition #1 and Condition #3, an immediate problem occurs. You are eating the same way you did for your whole life, but you have less ability to burn off these calories. The results? Any excess carbohydrates are converted to fat and stored.

Add in a slower metabolism (Condition #2) and you have the start of a nasty cycle. Without some significant change in nutrition or lifestyle, you have created the "fat gap". A more concise definition might read like this:

Fat Gap – noun; an increase in overall body fat despite a consistent pattern of diet and low-level exercise.

Here's another way to look at it. Let's say you weigh 150 pounds at age 45. Ten years later, when you are 55 years old, you still weigh 150 pounds.

You may say to yourself, "Hey, this is great. I haven't gained any weight in the past decade!"

While this is technically correct, you are, in fact, 5 pounds fatter!

You lost 5 pounds of muscle over the previous 10 years, but kept your body weight the same.

Guess what that over 5 pounds consists of?

Yup. Body fat.

Maintaining muscle mass is a constant battle! One we can NEVER stop fighting!

The upside is too powerful and the downside, too deadly.

We all have to do what we can to remain mobile and strong! Once you understand that this battle is never going away, it makes your path back to health that much clearer.

Fight on!

As mentioned earlier, we have managed to inject layers and layers of myths and outright lies into the topic of nutrition.

Nutrition can actually be remarkably simple. Together we can target your specific trouble spots and patterns.

There is a way.

You can get started here:

www.successfulaging.academy

Learn how to nourish yourself with the right food and eat with complete intention.

CHAPTER 8

WAKE UP CALL #2

Towards the beginning of this book, I told you the story of my near drowning and how it motivated me to both make changes in myself, and to help others through the Successful Aging Academy©.

Well, I have one final story for you.

This is the kind of story that solidified my dedication to you and your efforts to age successfully; and it confirms my beliefs about how some of my past decisions benefited me in a time of crisis.

This is a painful reminder of how everything can change in an instant…and yes, this story will make you cringe a bit.

We had lived in the same house for almost exactly 21 years, a long time by most any standard. Isn't it amazing what you can accumulate over time? We were all astounded by exactly how much there was to move, sell, throw away, donate, disperse to family, etc.

It was a huge job that had to be done, and it had a deadline.

I was fortunate since the new home I was moving to was available early, so I could start moving things in ahead of the actual possession date. This was proving to be a life-saver.

I had been moving, carrying, stacking and restacking things for weeks on end.

In the days and weeks leading up to "the event", I had carried nearly every piece of furniture you can imagine, twisted my body in clearly unhealthy ways, and generally pushed myself more than usual.

Again, this stuff just needed to get done.

To say that what happened next caught me off guard is an understatement. Big time!

It was Sunday, July 9th at about 6:45pm. I had been up since early that morning moving and packing, since we had sold our home and the closing date was now only days away.

I actually felt pretty good about where we were in the process compared to how much time remained. I felt we would be fine.

It was the end of a long day. I was extremely fatigued and dehydrated…and moving slowly.

"One more trip with the recycling bins, and I'll be done for the day", I thought to myself. I was spent.

So, I gathered up the big blue recycling bins, one atop the other, and headed down the short set of stairs into the garage.

This was a trip I had made – literally – thousands of times. But today was going to be different.

As I alternated my steps, I reached my right foot down to the bottom step, just above the landing. But…I missed calculated by an inch or two.

My heel grazed the bottom step, and instead planted all the way down to the bottom landing, missing the last step entirely.

It was awkward landing.

And then – in the blink of an eye – SNAP.

Instead of stopping, my body just kept going. There was no hesitation or resistance.

My body just kept dropping.

With my right leg giving way, all my body weight and the weight of the recycling in my arms, shifted over to my left leg - the one still trapped two steps back up the staircase.

SNAP number two...

Not good. I continued straight down.

The next thing I knew, I was on the garage floor.

One thing was *VERY* clear.

PAIN. Lots and lots of PAIN.

Let's just say I was shouting things I would not normally bring up in conversation. After a few moments of this, I tried to regain some composure.

"Hold on Art. Regroup here. Time to take inventory."

I felt both upper legs. No broken bones there. I ran my hands down each shin and wiggled my toes. Everything seemed OK there. I checked for blood or head injuries. Nothing.

I retrospect, I will admit one thing. I pretty much knew what had happened. Like when you recall a dream you had, right in the middle of the next day, for no apparent reason.

About half-way through the fall, I had one of those "moments of clarity".

"My knees are gone."

Sure enough. When I looked at my right kneecap, at first I thought I had displaced it; maybe knocked it off to the side.

My kneecap seemed to stick out...way out. The problem was, it really wasn't sticking out. It only looked that way because I had completely ruptured the very large quadriceps tendon that normally sits just above the kneecap.

With that gone, there was nothing but a bizarre empty space above my kneecap where a once-powerful tendon used to be...

My left knee had the same appearance.

I gave myself a diagnosis.

Complete rupture of BOTH quadriceps tendons.

And I knew I was right. And it all happened within seconds.

But wait, there's more...

So, there I am lying on the floor of my garage.

One of the first emotions to hit me was anger. I had blown out my left knee with a similar level of trauma 30 years earlier (almost to the week in fact).

And I will NEVER forget the pain I experienced once I woke up from surgery. It was FAR more painful than what I was experiencing at the moment.

Now, three decades later, I would have to face it again – times two!

The pain. The recovery process. All of it.

<u>But, this time I would be in my fifties. It was going to be a whole different ball game.</u>

I was livid, furious at my own stupidity for setting myself up for this.

(If this sounds familiar, yes, I felt as stupid as I had when I let myself get in my near drowning scenario!)

Then I got realistic. I needed to get to a hospital and get this whole process rolling. But, the only other person in earshot was my daughter, but she was asleep in her 2nd floor bedroom …with headphones on. And my cell phone was in my truck out in the driveway.

My plan?

In a seated position, I would shimmy along the garage floor backwards on my butt, out the garage door and around to the front of the house and somehow get my daughter's attention.

My quads were now pretty much in shock and, as strange as it seems, not causing me too much actual pain any more. This meant that once I got in position, it was just a matter of steady arm work.

At least I caught one break, so to speak. On my way out the garage door, I came across the four-wheel dolly I had been using to move the larger items. So I positioned my butt on the dolly and pushed myself along with my hands.

Once I made it to the front stairs, and after a few shouts didn't do the job, it was time to throw random items at my daughter's window.. stones, anything else I could reach.

To my credit, I went 3 for 3 hitting her window frame and she came down the stairs. Now the party could really get started.

Fifteen hours later I was in surgery. Facing 6 weeks of immobility before I could even start physical therapy.

Throughout this process, at least at the beginning, I kept notes on my milestones. Things like, moving from two crutches to one, showering again (that was a big day!), walking in my braces (thighs to ankles) a the near-by gym, etc.

I always had a goal to keep a few weeks ahead of where the doctors said I should be.

As of this writing, I am eight months into my recovery. I'm not at 100%, but I'm getting close. In fact, if we met face-to-face, and I didn't mention the surgery to you, it is unlikely you would be able to tell.

I learned a lesson or two. And I hope at least one of them will resonate with you.

Lesson #1: No matter what plans you have, no matter how busy you think life is, your health will dictate exactly what you will and will not do.

Neglect this and you invite disaster. You quickly learn that everything else is secondary to your health. Everything.

Every choice I made that day, in turn, made the outcome inevitable.

This was no accident. It wasn't some random accident that "happened to me" out of the blue.

I brought it about myself through poor decision making, and I paid the consequence.

I could not have planned it any more thoroughly.

Here's the analogy I make – What happened to me is a very condensed version of what many of us spend a lifetime doing.

We make poor decisions day after day.

These decisions accumulate over time.

In the end, we pay the consequences resulting in a loss of independence, poor quality of life, deteriorating health, etc.

Lesson #2: I keep myself in pretty good shape. I stay fairly lean and eat well. I work out regularly and as a general rule, make good choices about my health. This time I was actually MORE ready than I had been back when I nearly drowned.

No matter.

If you let yourself get too run down, too dehydrated, too stressed, etc. you open the door for accidents, or even professional and personal failures. That split second action, loss of focus or misstep that changes everything.

Had I had the focus to plant my foot squarely on the correct step, NONE of this happens. It's a non-story and I simply go about my day.

One second can change your world.

Listen to your body. Stop when you should. Rest when you need to. It will all get done.

However, by taking decent care of myself, my recovery was much quicker than many others who experienced similar injuries. The doctors confirmed it and, I knew it.

I have spoken with friends who went through the exact same injury and were in a wheelchair for months. After a full year, they were nowhere near fully recovered.

I am grateful my body still has the ability to recover well. However, I am fully aware that – just like the injury itself – I PLANNED that ability by taking certain steps ahead of time.

I was ready.

So I ask you…

What actions, thoughts, or choices do you make on a daily basis that you could change? Most likely in an instant…

Be mindful of the day to day issues that can stop or delay your steps to successful aging.

Attack them, one at a time! Take one step at a time until they are gone.

And start today!

Be READY for the challenge(s) we will ALL face when we least expect them!

Just like cooking, computers or virtually any other skill or trait, resiliency and 'mental strength' can be learned. It is NOT something only a few lucky ones are born with.

Find out how to create resiliency in your life, and then put it to use in ways you can now imagine.

www.successfulaging.academy

CONCLUSION

To sum up, here is my humble attempt to pull together ten actions to increase your lifespan, based upon research and observation. These actions are tied to various aspects of your life. This includes physical, spiritual/mental, social, cognitive, and nutritional qualities.

9 Actions to Help You Live Longer

1) **Run and walk quickly**. Studies have shown people who walk faster live longer. It's just that simple. When out walking, be mindful of your pace. If you find yourself slowing down, make a conscious effort to increase your speed.

2) **Learn constantly**. Always challenge the brain. The day you stop learning is the day you start to lose brain function. Cognitive skill is like any other physical trait; if you don't use it, you will lose it. Brain stimulating examples include: learning chess, doing the crossword

puzzle daily, reading or writing fiction or non-fiction outside your usual genre, attending a book reading or presentation/seminar, taking in a stage play or concert, traveling to a unique destination with a different culture, etc. Even learning a new physical skill impacts the brain in a positive way.

ABT = Always Be Thinking!

3) **Sleep restfully**. Human beings were designed for seven to eight hours of sleep. Those who get six or less hours of sleep per night, generally have a higher body weight than their counterparts. We now have a myriad of distractions available to us to keep us awake.

Calming the brain at the end of the day is the first step to better sleep. If you wake frequently, find the source of the disruption and research ways to overcome this. If you do not sleep restfully, you simply will not be firing on all cylinders.

In short, fix sleep first.

4) **Interact with others daily**. Be social and remain social. People with a vibrant social network are also shown to live longer than those in relative isolation. It is vital to get out of your comfort zone and interact with others.

5) **Eat colorfully and sparingly.** This requires some explanation. Your goal should be to eat a wide range

from the color palette; reds, greens, purples, etc. Work towards an entire assortment of colors.

This includes a wide range of fruits and vegetables. I have heard it phrased this way: "Avoid the white foods: bread, rice, cereal, pasta, crackers, etc." Refined foods tend to lack vibrant color, unless this color is artificially introduced.

The second part of the equation is to eat sparingly. Studies have shown that – up to a point - the less caloric intake you have, the longer you will live. In short, be aware of your portion sizes. In the US, this is perhaps one of the biggest contributors to the obesity epidemic.

NOTE: This does NOT apply to individuals whose caloric intake is already drastically low due to illness or frailty.

6) **Lift weights religiously**. Nothing has been shown to retain or even gain muscle mass better than resistance training, that's just a fact.

Running and walking won't do it and yoga won't do it. These activities have their place, but not as the sole source of exercise. It is important to realize that every year after the age of forty, you can lose up to a half pound of muscle mass per year. The only way to combat this atrophy is with resistance training.

7) **Worship and/or meditate regularly.** The inner peace that comes with these actions is a form of stress reduction. This is vital for a longer life and proper functioning. Whether you find contentment through Church, Tai Chi, Temple, or some other form of worship or meditation; attention to the needs of the 'soul', if you will, is vital for longevity.

8) **Stand up and lie down smoothly.** Move! Do so efficiently and often. In our modern lives, it is not uncommon to go entire days or even weeks with mobility limited to laying down, sitting in a chair, and standing up a few times, walking a little bit, perhaps navigating the occasional short flight of stairs and then laying down again.

   Studies have shown that people who have the mobility, agility, and relative body strength to go from a standing position down to a seated position on the floor, then get all the way back up smoothly with minimal support or excessive effort, live longer than those who struggle with this simple task. Stay mobile.

9) **Reduce all forms of inflammation, diligently.** More and more research is coming out saying that inflammation is at the center of many diseases; with links to Alzheimer's, heart disease, diabetes, and more.

The common link connects back to inflammation.

This does not mean take anti-inflammatory drugs constantly.

Investigate the list of foods which have an anti-inflammatory action in the body. Reducing inflammation can be accomplished through diet and exercise.

In fact, one of the primary nutritional approaches is a meal plan specifically designed to reduce your body's inflammation levels.

EPILOGUE

I have just spent roughly 100 pages presenting my thoughts on what it takes to age successfully.

Now what?

Well, first and foremost, **action is required**. Mindfulness of your own situation is vital.

Don't wake up some day and wonder what happened.

I nearly drowned before I realized I could no longer slide by on past physical abilities, fading innate skills, or wishful thinking.

If you went back in time and someone asked you at age twenty what your goals were, I'm guessing we would not hear this:

"When I get older I want to be overweight, feel like crap most of the time, be pretty much inactive, have no energy at all and no real plan for change."

Nobody set out with these as goals, but here we are. Only now you have some options. Change will not be easier to achieve next year or in 5 years.

Action is required now!

You are the disrupter.

You do so by stepping up and implementing a system.

Imagine having the confidence to approach – not just a health 'challenge' like weight loss – but ANY challenge, knowing full well how to break it down and DESTROY your "Big Rock".

No matter how intimidating it may appear at first.

You have the power of a real, psychological system behind you. Combine that with a community of people doing the EXACT same thing you are, and you become unstoppable!

Accountability has been missing for too many of us.

Now it has become an obligation.

Reach out, and we will work together to design your personal "Ideal You Project".

There is a very good reason the Phoenix is incorporated into the Successful Aging logo.

Stop for a moment and picture what your life would be like if you set your big, audacious goal…and then achieved it!

What would that include?

A lean physique?

Pain free joints?

The perfect companion?

An abundance of energy each and every day?

Living with a powerful purpose?

Complete, unshakable confidence that you could achieve any challenge you desired?

Your answers are your own. You shape your own future.

Contact the Successful Aging Academy today. Discover what it's all about and determine if you are a good fit.

www.successfulaging.academy

Complete the program and see what strength is on every level.

You are mobile and strong

You are resilient

You embrace action

You dictate your own future

You disrupt the status quo

You are a successful aging rebel

Are you ready?